Amino Acids – The Cure

Breaking Free: Overcoming Depression, Addictions, Obesity, and Anxiety Through Natural Amino Acid Therapy

By Rebecca Ricker

I0414205

Table of Contents

From helping to cure depression, addictions, anxiety and sexual issues to filling the complete nutritional requirements of both vegetarian and vegan diets, the significance of Amino Acids cannot be understated. With the added bonus of having absolutely no side effects whatsoever, the taking of these supplements without question form a win, win scenario.

And recent studies in the United States suggest that a cure for breast cancer, which is the second biggest killer of American women, could be as simple as adding Amino Acids to your diet.

With a complete list of the essential and non-essential Amino Acids, and the functions which they perform, this book will help to make it easy to spot what your body may require, to help you treat a wide variety of ailments.

Russell Burgess
Author

Chapter 1
The Importance of Amino Acids

My goal for this book is to impart to you the importance of amino acids and the danger to your body if amino acids are lacking in your diet. Amino acids are responsible for building and synthesizing vital proteins. Without them our body cannot survive. Amino acid therapy is one of the easiest ways to combat many health problems, but people seem very reluctant to try it. It may be that diet scams, snake oil salesmen, and other charlatans have made people wary of trying new or no-nonsense ways to improve their health. The question on everyone's lips, when presented with any kind of supplement, is "what are the side effects" and the answer is, in this case, none whatsoever. According to Dr. William Nelson, "Not only are there no side effects, but there are numerous side benefits. People with depression often find relief not only from depression but also insomnia, fatigue, GI symptoms, chronic pain, PMS, menopausal symptoms, obesity, food cravings, etc." This is revolutionary, to say the least. People need to understand that the body needs amino acids to function and in our society today, our diets are full of empty food which has been depleted by refined and over-processed ingredients. Amino acid therapy can help us improve our thinking processes so that we can make better food choices. Our diets have made us unable to think rationally or even process information correctly.

One of the problems found by dieters is the fact that no matter how much they diet they never lose very much weight and they feel horrible in the process. Many people come to the realization of this syndrome after several months of extreme exercises with very little, if any, body fat loss. Some people find themselves exercising for at least one hour a day, 6 days a week, and are exhausted and feel like they are fighting a losing battle. This is because their body has gone through too many "diet" scenarios, stress, malnutrition, and amino acid deficiency. In the book entitled "*The Diet Cure*" by Julia Ross, M. A., she goes into detail about what may be the cause of unexplained weight gain and depression.

In order to begin the process of healing, if you have any current medical issues, consult your doctor before adding these amino acids or supplements to your diet.

Chapter 2
The Road To Wellness

The first things to incorporate are the amino acid supplements listed below as well as complete B vitamins, magnesium, calcium, zinc, and vitamin E. Just the addition of the following minimum doses of amino acids will give you great hope:

L-Glutamine, 500mg (stops cravings, enhances relaxation) (before breakfast, mid morning, mid afternoon)

L-tyrosine, 500mg (energizing, mental focus) (before breakfast, mid morning, mid afternoon)

DLPA (DL-phenylalanine), 500mg (comfort, pleasure, reduce pain) (before breakfast, mid morning, mid afternoon)

GABA, 100-500mg (to de-stress, relax) (mid morning, mid afternoon, bedtime)

5-HTP, 50mg (improve mood, sleep, and evening cravings) (mid morning, mid afternoon, bedtime)

You should begin with the minimum dosages to make sure that you don't have any adverse reactions.

The amino acids mentioned previously are very important components to get us started on the road to wellness. L-Glutamine, L-tyrosine, DL-phenylalanine, GABA, and 5-HTP are the starter kit needed to begin to think clearly, feel better and have enough energy to move on to the next part of the program. This part includes getting a complete amino acid supplement, such as **Optimal Amino Blend by Seeking Health.** There are many choices for Amino Acid supplements out there but this product is vegetarian, offers all of the amino acids, have no soy products within them, and they are gluten free. Now lets move on to what these complete amino acid supplements have to offer us.

The essentials are: histidine, isoleucine, leucine, lysine, methionine, phenylalanine, threonine, tryptophan, and valine.

Histidine promotes stomach digestive secretions, helps in the production of red blood cells, strengthens nerve receptors in the inner ear, improves the function and keeps the nerve cells in the inner ear healthy.

Isoleucine reduces stress, helps us to think clearly, and is a vital source of energy for our muscles.

Leucine stabilizes blood sugar levels, promotes healing in the skin and bones, and produces energy.

Lysine forms collagen, has an energizing affect, improves stress tolerance, inhibits virus growth, builds antibodies, and, most important to me, improves fat metabolism.

Methionine promotes antibody production, prevents hair loss, prevents excessive fat buildup in the liver, and regenerates cells in the liver and kidney.

Phenylalanine elevates positive mood, alertness, ambition, and enhances memory and learning.

Theonine improves digestion, absorption of nutrients, and food assimilation.

Tryptophan is a mood regulator which has a calming effect, helps to burn body fat by stimulating the release of growth hormones, and reduces carbohydrate cravings.

Valine is responsible for muscle coordination, stabilizing emotions, mental vigor, and promoting restful sleep.

Here is the complete list of **Essential Amino Acids** and the functions:

Amino
Acetyl-L-carnitine (to induce a pleasant visual and mental clarity, improves long-term memory and learning ability. Improves insulin response.) Studies have shown that a combination of Acetyl-L-carnitine and lipoic acid enhance brain energy, helping to improve mood and reduce the effects of age-associated memory impairment.
DLPA (DL-phenylalanine) (comfort, pleasure, reduce pain) (Phenylalanine stimulates the thyroid gland and is used by the gland to make thyroxine (a hormone involved in the regulation of metabolism and heat production) and by the brain to stimulate production of adrenaline and noradrenaline, used by the body to react to stress.)
GABA or GABA w/taurine and glycine, (to de-stress and relax muscles)
5-HTP 5HTP is a byproduct of tryptophan. 5-HTP works in the brain and central nervous system by increasing the production of the chemical serotonin. 5-HTP is used for sleep disorders, depression, anxiety, migraine and tension-type headaches, fibromyalgia, binge eating associated with obesity, premenstrual syndrome (PMS), premenstrual dysphoric disorder (PMDD), and attention deficit-hyperactivity disorder (ADHD). (improve mood, sleep, and evening cravings)
L-Histidine Histidine is important in the production of red and white blood cells. It strengthens the nerve receptors in the inner ear, nourishes the nerve cells of the hearing mechanism, and improves the function of the auditory nerve. Histidine promotes stomach digestive secretions, is an excellent carrier for iron and zinc, and promotes normal sexual response.
L-Lysine Lysine promotes bone growth by helping to form collagen, cartilage, and other connective tissues. It aids in calcium absorption, promotes insulin production, improves the uptake of branched-chain amino acids -- valine, isoleucine, and leucine -- in muscle, increases protein synthesis, and has an anti fatigue effect. Improves stress tolerance and

fat metabolism, inhibits the growth of viruses and builds antibodies. L-Lysine is an essential amino acid which acts as a precursor for several other amino acids, including L-Citrulline (needed in the body for normal protein metabolism) and L-carnitine (needed for fat metabolism). L-Lysine is crucial for the formation of collagen, a major part of the body's connective tissues. L-Lysine also contributes to energy production when converted to acetyl coenzyme A, one of the principal fuels for the Krebs cycle.

L-Methionine

(It is required for liver health and detoxification, prevents fat buildup in the liver, helps regenerate liver and kidney cells, and promotes antibody production.)

L-Ornithine

Ornithine stimulates hormones, such as insulin. It decreases body fat, strengthens the immune system, promotes healing, promotes liver function and regeneration, and is important for detoxifying ammonia.

L-Tryptophan

Mood, Relaxation, Sleep

The essential amino acid L-Tryptophan helps support relaxation, restful sleep and feeling better. It plays a part in the synthesis of both melatonin and serotonin, hormones involved with mood and stress response. L-Tryptophan also supports immune functions because it is the body's precursor to the kynurenines that regulate immunity. If needed, L-Tryptophan converts to niacin in the body, which supports circulation, a healthy nervous system, the metabolism of food, and the production of hydrochloric acid for the digestive system. Source Naturals L-Tryptophan is extremely pure and is regularly tested to ensure the highest standards of quality.

Theanine

Neurotransmitter

Promotes Relaxation and Learning Ability

Theanine is a unique amino acid found almost exclusively in green tea that exerts beneficial effects on brain metabolism. Theanine induces relaxation without causing drowsiness, as measured by increased generation of alpha-waves. Theanine may improve learning ability and sensations of pleasure by affecting dopamine and serotonin neurotransmitters in the brain. Also, Theanine exerts protective effects on the brain by antagonizing glutamate toxicity. Jarrow Formulas Theanine 100 is 100% L-theanine, made enzymatically from amino acids and is identical to the theanine found in green tea.

We spoke about essential amino acids, now we will talk about the nonessential amino acids and their functions. Nonessential amino acids are made in the body, but if there is a lack of essential amino acids the nonessential amino acids cannot be synthesized correctly. This is why it is so important, when you are on the road to wellness, that you incorporate all of the amino acids, essential and nonessential, in supplement form until your body begins to recover.

Nonessential Amino Acids	What is their function?
Alanine	Fuel for the brain, nervous system, and muscles
Arginine	Stimulates the release of growth hormone, decreases body fat, improves tissue healing, increases collagen, and stimulates the immune system.
Aspartic Acid	Increases activity in the central nervous system, helps fatigue resistance, increases stamina, increases endurance, produces energy, strengthens the immune system, and protects the liver
Citrulline	Stimulates the immune system, detoxifies, and helps the body recover from fatigue
Cysteine	Aggressively scavenges free radicals, prevents cell damage from cigarette smoke, detoxifies, promotes healing, helps in carbohydrate metabolism
Glutamic Acid	Brain metabolism, brain fuel, transports potassium across the blood brain barrier, helps the brain to detoxify, metabolizes sugars and fats
Glutamine	Brain metabolism, energy for the brain, reduces the loss of potassium and sodium electrolytes
Glycine	Essential for muscle function, breaks down glycogen and frees energy, builds immune system, calms the brain and nerves
Ornithine	Stimulates the release of growth hormone, decreases body fat, promotes healing, increases muscle mass, promotes liver function regeneration

Proline	Promotes growth and function of tendons, joints, joint linings, and heart muscles, stores energy, essential component of collagen
Serine	Energy storage, builds immune system, produces antibodies, supports skin metabolism
Taurine	Development of fetal brain and central nervous system, body manufacture this from methionine and cystine, moderates cholesterol production and fat metabolism, improves digestion, improves intestine disorders, prevents cardiac loss of potassium
Tyrosine	Precursor of thyroid and adrenal hormones, important to the function of adrenal, pituitary and thyroid glands, brain stimulant, mood elevator, responsible for pigmentation of the skin and hair, stimulates growth hormone, reduces body fat, generates red and white blood cells

Chapter 3
Amino Acids and Cancer

Cancer in the United States has reached an alarming number of our population. The highest incidence and type of cancer reported, according to the CDC, is breast cancer http://apps.nccd.cdc.gov/uscs/statevsnational.aspx . This is alarming to say the least. Breast cancer is also reported as the second highest killer of American women. So what can we do about it? Well, a recent study done by the Center For Integrated Protein Science in Munich states that the cure could be as easy as amino acid therapy. The research showed that the amino acids L-phenylalanine, L-tyrosine, and tryptophan was effective in inhibiting cancer cell growth in a permanent manner. This is astounding evidence that amino acids are absolutely essential to cancer prevention and longevity.

To know that these simple amino acids L-phenylalanine, L-tyrosine, and tryptophan, can make such a difference in the prevention of breast cancer should give us pause to find out what they are and which foods contain them. Of course, supplementation is a good option especially for vegans or vegetarians and with our food supply somewhat depleted it is always a good practice to supplement to be sure you are getting these important nutrients.

Phenylalanine is an essential amino acid found in eggs (highest concentration), beef, lamb, fish, turkey, cottage cheese, seaweed, watercress, kidney beans, spinach (cooked), turnip greens, broccoli raab, and peanuts. It is responsible for stimulating the thyroid gland and making thyroxin, which regulates metabolism and heat production, and stimulates adrenaline and noradrenalin production in the brain. Phenylalanine is involved in the production of neurotransmitters which control the impulse transmissions between nerve cells and dopamine transmission, sustain an improved and cheerful mood, increases focus and ambition, increases learning and memory.

Tyrosine is an amino acid which also plays an important role in the thyroid, pituitary, and adrenal hormones. It is also responsible for elevated mood as well as the production of melanin which is responsible for hair and skin pigmentation, stimulating the release of growth hormone, and generating red and white blood cells. Tyrosine can be found in seaweed, eggs, cottage cheese, fish, turkey, mustard greens, pork, cream cheese, chicken, duck, peanuts, kidney beans, cooked spinach, watercress, mustard greens, and sesame seeds.

Tryptophan is an amino acid which is instrumental in the production of the neurotransmitter serotonin. Serotonin is responsible for mood regulation and creates a calming effect. Tryptophan also aids in the assimilation of vitamin B complex, releases growth hormone, reduces carbohydrate cravings, and promotes smooth muscle growth[1]. Tryptophan can be found in seaweed, eggs, sesame seeds, duck, turkey, quail, squab, fish, shrimp, lobster, crab, goat, watercress, oat bran, chia seeds, spinach, watercress, crimini mushrooms, turnip greens, broccoli raab, parsley, and asparagus.

Chapter 4
Amino Acids and Addictions

Now we will explore addiction and how most addictions are caused by biological imbalances. There is much research on the causes of addiction, but at this time the most widely used prescription for addictions is the different "Anonymous" groups; Alcoholics Anonymous, Narcotics Anonymous, Cocaine Anonymous, Marijuana Anonymous, and a host of others are all trying to solve the problem of addiction from a 12 step program perspective. There is scientific proof that the cause of addiction is more than just behavioral and is biological. Research has shown that L-Glutamine, GABA (gabapentin), and proper nutrition is instrumental in helping patients become free of addictions to drugs, alcohol, cigarettes and any other substances, within a three week period of time.

Alcoholics Anonymous, Narcotics Anonymous, Cocaine Anonymous, Marijuana Anonymous, and a host of others are all noble attempts to cure addiction from a 12 step program perspective, but the fact is that there is scientific proof that the cause of addiction is more than just behavioral and is in fact biological. By looking at the effects of these biological imbalances in an addict and adding proper nutrients, the cravings for the addictive substance can be completely halted. This comes from research studies done by Julia Ross (2008) and many other psychologists and physicians in the specific field of addiction. The substance abuse and addictions studied include alcohol, marijuana, cocaine, speed, opiates, tobacco, and prescription drugs.

Historically, anonymous groups have been the only option for substance abusers to turn to. This has worked for some, but the majority of people who have trouble with substance abuse go from one substance to another to try to take care of their cravings. Alcohol and drug treatment centers, such as the one in San Francisco where Ross (2008) practiced, who use anonymous groups and prescription drugs to curb the substance abuse, find that 80% to 90% of all clients would relapse back into their addiction. Most alcoholics and drug users will substitute the addictive substance with sweets and refined foods because, as Ross points out, "sugar is almost identical to alcohol biochemically. Both are highly refined, simple carbohydrates and are instantly absorbed... skyrocket*ing* blood sugar levels and temporarily raise potent mood chemicals in the brain." Chastain (2006) states that the pharmacological approach to the treatment of alcoholism are the drugs Disulfiram, Naltrexone, Acamprosate, Tiapride, and Naranjo which have serious side effects including "nausea, vomiting, pounding in the chest, decrease in blood pressure," sedation, sleeplessness, excessive sweating, tremor, headache, and Disulfiram has been known to produce hepatitis. This study also showed the effects of alcohol on the protein molecules in the brain; alcohol has a detrimental effect on neurotransmitter activity in the brain (Chastain). Head (2006) shows that the use of traditional medicine, used to alleviate problems caused by addictions, only mask the symptoms and at times actually cause addiction to the medication used to help stop the initial addiction. Many of these pharmaceutical drugs are used to increase serotonin in the brain which has been noted is depleted in most addiction patients.

A study done by Blum et al. (1990) illustrates that experimentation done on humans and animals prove that nutrient deficiencies can be the cause of addiction and hinder the recovery of addicts. These deficiencies have caused a deficit in the neurotransmitters serotonin, dopamine, and GABA (Blum et al.). Serotonin, as stated by Fusar-Poli et al. (2007), has been implicated in a wide variety of functions such as mood, anxiety, sleep, aggression, and sexual and cognitive functions. As study done by Kapus et al. (2008) showed that anxiety disorders, in mice and in humans, are caused by a lack of serotonin in the brain. The use of GABA can lead to a safer therapeutic approach to anxiety disorders than the use of narcotic approaches or sedatives. A study done by Markus et al. (2008) showed that serotonin levels increased with the use of tryptophan which elevated overall mood and sense of well being in the study group. A study done by Fusar-Poli et al (2007) showed that tryptophan is the precursor to serotonin and the lack of tryptophan has noticeable effects on serotonin levels in the brain.

utritional supplement which Ross (2008) suggests would increase serotonin levels in the brain include L-tryptophan, 5-HTP, St. Johns Wort, Melatonin and vitamin B6 (p.3). Blum et al. (1990) established similar results in their study which stated that supplementation of the amino acid L-tryptophan converts to serotonin in the brain. Markus et al. (2008) also concluded that the use of tryptophan sources were advantageous to the availability of essential amino acids to brain chemistry. Fusar-Poli et al. (2007) also concurred that the lack of tryptophan had a significant lowered effect in the brain activity which is normally present in happy individuals. Supplementation with L-tryptophan, 5-HTP, St. Johns Wort, Melatonin, and Vitamin B-6 is just one way to increase serotonin levels in the brain to bring about recovery from addictions. Diet can play a major role in raising serotonin levels as well. According to Ross (1999) whole food carbohydrates can raise serotonin levels in the brain and give the needed nutrients to fuel the body. Ross (2008) states that food items which naturally raise serotonin levels are 25-30 grams of good quality protein per meal; this includes eggs, chicken, cottage cheese, and red meat. Low starch green, yellow, red, and purple vegetables, avocados, olive oil, coconut milk, coconut oil, nuts and seeds, fruit, squash, beans, potatoes, rice and corn. The foods to avoid are sweets, white flour products, caffeine, sugar substitutes, and fried foods . Diet alone can raise serotonin levels, but studies have shown that serotonin will also rise naturally after doing moderate exercise outdoors (Ross, 1999).

Fusar-Poli et al. (2007) points out that psychological problems stem from depletion, or low levels, of essential chemicals in the brain. These psychological problems can manifest themselves as depression, anxiety disorders, sleep disorders, aggressive behaviors, and lack of sexual and cognitive functions. The chemicals which control these functions are serotonin, endorphins, dopamine, norepinephrine, gamma-amino-butyric acid (GABA), and opioid systems in the brain.

The addition of essential amino acid supplementation is highly useful in alleviating these psychological problems, which are the symptoms of low levels of essential chemicals in the brain. One study done by Pålsson et al. (2007) showed that the amino acid L-arginine could have therapeutic effects on the cognitive dysfunctions in schizophrenia. The study shows that these amino acids could be used to alleviate the problems associated with drug use and schizophrenia. Also, in this study, L-lysine was shown to protect mice from the effects of PCP. The study done by Blum et al. (1990) showed that the amino acids L-phenylalanine and L-tyrosine convert to dopamine and norepinephrine; and L-glutamine converts to GABA. A study done by Porter et al. (2007) showed the positive effects of the amino acid tryptophan on cortisol in saliva. The participants in the study were elderly individuals who had recently recovered from depression and healthy elderly. The study was done using two amino acid mixtures; one which contained tryptophan and one which did not contain tryptophan. The study showed a definite difference in the positive effects of tryptophan on depression.

Nutrition therapy is an emerging successful alternative to traditional substance abuse therapy and offers people suffering from substance abuse real and lasting relief from the substance abuse prison. The detoxification process can be painful and cause many substance abusers to think twice about going through the pain of quitting. According to Chastain (2006) "Excessive glutamate activity, during withdrawal, contributes to cell death and thus frequent withdrawal may lead to irreversible alcoholic brain damage." It is also interesting to note that "chronic alcohol use leads to reduced brain levels of endorphin, which contribute to the negative emotional states that accompany alcoholic withdrawal." This is where nutrition therapy comes into play in the form of several essential amino acids.

A study done by Crokford, White, and Campbell (2001) showed that supplementing with GABA was instrumental in helping the patient become free of the addiction to benzodiazepine, as well as cigarettes and any other substances, within a three week period of time. The result also showed that using GABA left no withdrawal symptoms as the patient went off the addictive substances. Crokford et al. goes on to state that "It has been reported *that GABA is* helpful in the management of pain syndromes, anxiety, and alcohol withdrawal." A study done by Gass and Olive (2008) shows that treating cocaine use by supplementing with the amino acid L-cysteine can reduce cravings, withdrawals, and relapse in patients. The study also showed that after a four week period of time the results showed that L-cysteine was still instrumental in reducing or alleviating all cravings and withdrawals in these patients.

According to Head (2006) the use of Alpha-lipoic acid, amino acids acetyl-L-carnitine, L-arginine, L-glutamine, taurine, N-acetylcysteine and other supplements are instrumental in the alleviation of addictions, are typically without side effects, and address nutrient deficiencies, oxidative stress, and other etiologieal factors. A study done by Roberts (2005), shows the effectiveness of GABA on addictions; specifically cocaine addiction. The positive results from this study have prompted studies on humans to see if GABA has the same positive effect on lessening or completely alleviating the cravings and withdrawals associated with addictions. In studies done by Ross (2008) all addictions were alleviated by the use of supplemental L-tryptophan, L-tyrosine, GABA, DL-phenalanine, and L-glutamine. The specific use of L-glutamine has shown significant results in alleviating cravings of addictive substances.

Conclusion

In conclusion, we now know that there is scientific proof that the cause of addiction, and many other illnesses, is more than just behavioral and is in fact biological. By looking at the studies and the conclusions of the studies, the effects of these biological imbalances in an individual and by adding proper nutrients, the illnesses and symptoms can be completely halted. The lack of proper nutrition is a significant reason for these illnesses. There are no known side effects to the use of amino acids as a tool in nutritional therapy, which makes supplementation, using amino acids, a wonderful tool to the road to optimal health.

The End

Bibliography

Blum, K., Rassner, M., & Payne, J E (August 1990). Neuro-nutrient therapy for compulsive disease: rationale and clinical evidence. (physiological aspects of alcoholism). *Addiction & Recovery*, 10, n2. p. 12(5). Retrieved September 11, 2010, from Academic OneFile via Gale: http://find.galegroup.com.ezproxy.liberty.edu:2048/gtx/start.do?prodId=A ONE&userGroupName=vic_liberty

Chastain, G. (2006). Alcohol, Neurotransmitter Systems, and Behavior. *The Journal of General Psychology*, *133*(4), 329-35. Doi: 10.3200/GENP.133.4.329-335

Crockford, D., White, W., & Campbell, B. (2001). Gabapentin use in benzodiazepine dependence and detoxification. *Canadian Journal Of Psychiatry. Revue Canadienne De Psychiatrie*, *46*(3), 287. Retrieved from MEDLINE with Full Text database.

Fusar-Poli, P., Allen, P., Lee, F., Surguladze, S., Tunstall, N., Y Fu, C. H., Brammer, M. J., Cleare, A. J., & McGuire, P. K. (2007). Modulation of neural response to happy and sad faces by acute tryptophan depletion. Psychopharmacology, 193(1), 31-44. Retrieved August 23, 2010, from ProQuest Psychology Journals. (Document ID: 1290835021).

Gass, J., & Olive, M. (2008). Glutamatergic substrates of drug addiction and alcoholism. *Biochemical Pharmacology*, *75*(1), 218-265. doi:10.1016/j.bcp.2007.06.039.

Giese, C., Lepthien, S., Metzner, L., Brandsch, M., Budisa, N. and Lilie, H. (2008), Intracellular uptake and inhibitory activity of aromatic fluorinated amino acids in human breast cancer cells. ChemMedChem, 3: 1449–1456. doi: 10.1002/cmdc.200800108

Head, K. (2006). Peripheral Neuropathy: Pathogenic Mechanisms and Alternative Therapies. *Alternative Medicine Review*, *11*(4), 294-329. Retrieved from Academic Search Complete database.

Hunter, B. (2006) *A Whole Foods Primer.* Basic Health Publications, Inc. Laguna Beach, CA.

Kapus, G., Gacsályi, I., Vegh, M., Kompagne, H., Hegedus, E., Leveleki, C., Hársing, L., Barkóczy, J., Bilkei-gorzó, A., & Lévay, G. (2008). Antagonism of AMPA receptors produces anxiolytic-like behavior in rodents: Effects of GYKI 52466 and its novel analogues. Psychopharmacology, 198(2), 231-41. Retrieved August 23, 2010, from

Markus, C., Firk, C., Gerhardt, C., Kloek, J., & Smolders, G.. (2008). Effect of different tryptophan sources on amino acids availability to the brain and mood in healthy volunteers. Psychopharmacology, 201(1), 107-14. Retrieved August 23, 2010, from ProQuest Psychology Journals. (Document ID: 1579240641).

Nelson, William, NMD Article Source: http://EzineArticles.com/19902

Pålsson, E., Fejgin, K., Wass, C., Engel, J., Svensson, L., & Klamer, D. (2007). The amino acid l-lysine blocks the disruptive effect of phencyclidine on prepulse inhibition in mice. *Psychopharmacology, 192*(1), 9-15. doi:10.1007/s00213-006-0683-x.

Porter, R. J., Gallagher, P., & O'Brien, J. T. (2007). Effects of rapid tryptophan depletion on salivary cortisol in older people recovered from depression, and the healthy elderly. Journal of Psychopharmacology, 21(1), 71-75. Retrieved August 23, 2010, from ProQuest Psychology Journals. (Document ID: 1268367181).

Roberts, D. (2005). Preclinical evidence for GABA.sub.B agonists as a pharmacotherapy for cocaine addiction. *Physiology & Behavior, 86*(1/2), 18-20. doi:10.1016/j.physbeh.2005.06.017.

Ross, J. (1999). The diet cure. Penguin Publishers, New York, NY.

Ross, J. (2008). Presentation given on Neuro-nutrient Therapy: 21st century treatment for addictive disorders. San Diego, Ca.

www.ingramcontent.com/pod-product-compliance
Lightning Source LLC
Chambersburg PA
CBHW061942280526
45787CB00004B/1694